5-MUNITE CORE EXERCISE FOR BEGINNERS

A Journey to Strength, Balance, and Vitality

Julius Theobald

Disclaimer Statement

Please keep in mind that the contents of this booklet are meant for educational and recreational purposes. Every effort has been made to offer accurate, up-to-date, reliable, and thorough information. There are, however, no stated or implied assurances of any kind. Readers understand that the author is providing competent counsel. The content in this book originates from several sources. Please seek the opinion of a competent professional before using any of the tactics outlined in this book. By reading this book, the reader agrees that the author will not be held accountable for any direct or indirect damages resulting from the use of the information contained therein, including, but not limited to, errors, omissions, or inaccuracies.

Table of Contents

INTRODUCTION

Welcome, dear reader, to the vibrant world of "5-Minute Core Exercises for Beginners" Before you dive into the invigorating sea of core workouts, let me extend a warm, virtual handshake and a pat on the back. You've taken the first step towards a stronger, healthier you, and that deserves a round of applause!

Now, let's take a moment to acknowledge something crucial: embarking on a fitness journey, especially one targeting your core, can be both exciting and daunting. Trust me, I've been there. Picture this: you've decided it's time to sculpt those abs, tone those oblique's, and strengthen that lower back. You're pumped, you're ready, but then reality hits, life is busy, time is short, and suddenly, the idea of squeezing in a workout feels about as feasible as mastering quantum physics in five minutes.

But fear not, my fellow core crusaders! This book is your beacon of hope in the stormy sea of fitness confusion. Whether you're a total newbie to the world of core workouts or someone who's dabbled but never quite found their groove, consider this your roadmap to success. Think of me as your trusty guide, your fitness confidant, and occasional cheerleader, here to sprinkle a bit of humor and a whole lot of empathy into your journey.

So, why the focus on core exercises, you might ask? Well, let me tell you, it's not just about getting that coveted six-pack (although hey, that's a nice bonus!). Strengthening your core is like laying a solid foundation for a skyscraper, you wouldn't build a towering structure on shaky ground, would you? Your core is your body's powerhouse, the epicenter of strength and stability. From lifting groceries to perfecting your yoga poses to simply sitting up straight, a strong core impacts every aspect of your daily life.

But hey, I get it, finding the time and motivation to work on your core can feel like trying to solve a Rubik's Cube blindfolded. That's why I've crafted this book with your busy schedule and wavering motivation levels in mind. We're talking bite-sized workouts that you can sneak in while waiting for your morning coffee to brew or during those commercial breaks of your favorite TV show. Yes, you heard me right, no more excuses about not having enough time. If you can spare five minutes (and let's face it, we all waste more time scrolling through cat memes on the internet), you can crush a core workout.

Now, before we dive into the nitty-gritty of planks, crunches, and all things core-related, let me assure you of something, I understand where you're coming from. I know the struggle of trying to squeeze into those workout clothes that seem to have mysteriously shrunk overnight (spoiler alert: they didn't). I know the frustration of staring at your reflection in the gym mirror, wondering if you'll ever see any progress. And I know the temptation of hitting the snooze button instead of hitting the gym.

But here's the thing, every journey, no matter how daunting it may seem, begins with a single step. And you, my friend, have already taken that step simply by picking up this book. So give yourself a pat on the back, maybe do a little victory dance (I won't judge), and get ready to embark on a journey that's as rewarding as it is sweaty.

Throughout these pages, you'll find everything you need to kick start your core transformation. From understanding the anatomy of your core to mastering proper form and technique, we've got you covered. And hey, if you ever find yourself struggling or feeling overwhelmed, just remember, I've got your back (pun intended).

So, without further ado, let's turn the page and begin this adventure together. Get ready to feel the burn, laugh at my corny jokes, and emerge on the other side stronger, fitter, and maybe even with a newfound love for core workouts.

Here's to stronger cores and brighter days ahead!

Warmest regards,

GETTING STARTED

Embarking on a journey to strengthen your core is an admirable decision, one that can significantly impact your overall health and well-being. In this chapter, we'll delve into the essential steps to get started with core exercises. From assessing your current fitness level to setting realistic goals and creating a consistent routine, we'll lay the groundwork for your core transformation.

Assessing Your Current Fitness Level

Before diving headfirst into a new exercise regimen, it's essential to take stock of where you currently stand in terms of fitness. This step not only helps you understand your starting point but also enables you to tailor your workouts to suit your abilities and avoid injury.

Start by evaluating your endurance, strength, and flexibility. Can you hold a plank for more than a few seconds, or do you struggle to maintain proper form? Can you perform a full set of crunches without feeling fatigued, or do you find yourself struggling midway through? These are the questions to ponder as you assess your current fitness level.

Next, consider any existing health conditions or injuries that may affect your ability to engage in certain exercises. If you have back pain, for example, you'll want to choose core exercises that are gentle on your spine, such as pelvic tilts or seated core rotations. Consulting with a healthcare professional or a certified fitness trainer can provide valuable insights into how to navigate these challenges safely.

Remember, there's no shame in starting small. Everyone has to begin somewhere, and progress is measured not by where you start but by how far you've come. So, be honest with yourself about your current abilities, and approach your workouts with patience and self-compassion.

Setting Realistic Goals

With a clear understanding of your current fitness level, it's time to set realistic goals that will guide your core exercise journey. Goals serve as the roadmap to your destination, providing direction and motivation along the way. However, it's essential to set goals that are both achievable and meaningful to you.

Start by identifying what you hope to accomplish through your core workouts. Do you want to improve your posture, alleviate back pain, or sculpt a defined six-pack? Your goals should reflect your personal aspirations and priorities.

Once you've clarified your objectives, break them down into smaller, manageable milestones. For example, if your ultimate goal is to hold a plank for two minutes straight, you might set intermediate goals of increasing your plank duration by 15 seconds each week.

It's also crucial to make your goals smart, specific, measurable, attainable, relevant, and time-bound. Instead of saying, "I want to get stronger," try setting a goal like, "I will increase my plank hold time from 30 seconds to one minute within four weeks." This gives you a clear target to aim for and allows you to track your progress effectively.

Above all, be flexible with your goals and willing to adjust them as needed. Fitness is a journey filled with twists and turns, and sometimes, unexpected obstacles may arise. By staying adaptable and resilient, you'll be better equipped to overcome challenges and stay on course toward your ultimate objectives.

Creating a Consistent Routine

Consistency is the cornerstone of any successful fitness program, and core exercises are no exception. Without regular practice, you'll struggle to see significant improvements in strength, endurance, or appearance. That's why it's crucial to establish a consistent workout routine that fits seamlessly into your lifestyle.

Begin by scheduling dedicated time for core workouts in your weekly calendar. Treat these appointments with the same level of importance as you would a meeting or appointment, you wouldn't cancel on your boss, so don't cancel on yourself!

When selecting a time for your workouts, consider your natural energy levels and preferences. Some people prefer to exercise first thing in the morning to kick start their day, while others find it more convenient to squeeze in a workout during their lunch break or in the evening after work. Choose a time that feels right for you and commit to it wholeheartedly.

In addition to setting aside specific time slots for exercise, it's essential to vary your routine to prevent boredom and plateauing. Incorporate a mix of core exercises targeting different muscle groups, such as planks, crunches, Russian twists, and leg raises. This not only keeps your workouts interesting but also ensures that you're engaging all aspects of your core for comprehensive strength development.

Lastly, don't forget to listen to your body and prioritize rest and recovery. Overtraining can lead to burnout, injury, and diminished performance, so be sure to give yourself adequate time to rest and recharge between workouts. Remember, progress isn't just about how hard you push yourself, it's also about how well you take care of yourself outside the gym.

By assessing your current fitness level, setting realistic goals, and creating a consistent routine, you'll lay a solid foundation for your core exercise journey. So, lace up your sneakers, grab a water bottle, and get ready to embark on a transformative adventure toward a stronger, healthier you. The journey won't always be easy, but trust me—it'll be worth it in the end

CORE ANATOMY BASICS

Understanding the anatomy of your core is like having a map to navigate through a dense forest, it provides clarity, direction, and insight into how your body functions. In this chapter, we'll delve into the intricacies of core anatomy, exploring the muscles that make up this vital area, understanding their functionality, and debunking common myths surrounding core strength.

Exploring the Core Muscles

When most people think of the core, they envision six-pack abs and toned oblique's. While these muscles certainly play a significant role in core strength, the core encompasses a much broader network of muscles than meets the eye. To truly understand the complexity of the core, we must explore its anatomy from the inside out.

At the center of the core lies the powerhouse known as the transverse abdominis. This deep-lying muscle wraps around the torso like a corset, providing stability and support to the spine and pelvis. Think of it as your body's natural weightlifting belt, engaging to brace the core during movements like lifting, twisting, and bending.

Surrounding the transverse abdominis are the internal and external oblique's, which run diagonally along the sides of the torso. These muscles play a crucial role in rotational movements and lateral stability, helping you twist and turn with ease while maintaining proper alignment. Moving outward, we encounter the rectus abdominis, more commonly known as the "six-pack" muscles. While aesthetically pleasing, the primary function of the rectus abdominis is spinal flexion, allowing you to curl forward and sit up from a lying position.

Finally, we have the multifidus, erector spinae, and quadratus lumbered, which form the back extensor muscles of the core. These muscles work in tandem with the abdominals to provide balance, support, and protection to the spine, helping you maintain an upright posture and resist forces that could cause injury.

Understanding the intricate interplay between these muscles is essential for developing a well-rounded core exercise routine. By targeting all aspects of the core from the deep stabilizers to the superficial movers you'll build a foundation of strength and stability that extends far beyond mere aesthetics.

Understanding Core Functionality

Now that we've identified the key players in the core orchestra, let's explore how these muscles work together to perform everyday movements and maintain spinal health. At its core (pun intended), the primary function of the core is to provide stability and support to the spine and pelvis, allowing for efficient movement and load-bearing activities.

Imagine your core as the sturdy trunk of a tree, anchoring your limbs and allowing them to move with precision and control. Whether you're bending down to tie your shoes, lifting groceries off the ground, or simply sitting up straight in your chair, your core is constantly engaged to maintain proper alignment and prevent injury.

One of the core's most important functions is spinal stabilization, particularly during dynamic movements like walking, running, and lifting. The transverse abdominis acts as a natural weightlifting belt, cinching around the waist to create intra-abdominal pressure and support the spine under load.

Additionally, the oblique's and back extensors work synergistically to resist rotational forces and maintain lateral stability, preventing excessive twisting or bending of the spine. This stability is essential for protecting the delicate structures of the spine and reducing the risk of injury during physical activity.

Beyond its role in movement and stability, the core also plays a vital role in posture and balance. A strong, stable core provides a solid foundation for the rest of the body, allowing you to maintain an upright posture and move with grace and efficiency.

Understanding the functionality of the core goes beyond knowing the names of its constituent muscles it's about appreciating the intricate choreography that occurs with every movement you make. By cultivating awareness and mindfulness of your core, you'll not only enhance your physical performance but also reduce the risk of injury and improve your overall quality of life.

Common Core Strength Myths Debunked

In the quest for a stronger, more defined core, it's easy to fall prey to common misconceptions and myths surrounding core strength training. Let's debunk some of these myths and set the record straight once and for all.

- **Myth #1:** Crunches are the key to six-pack abs. While crunches can certainly help strengthen the rectus abdominis and create definition in the midsection, they're not the be-all and end-all of core training. In fact, focusing exclusively on crunches can neglect other important aspects of core strength, such as stability and functional movement patterns. Instead of fixating on crunches, incorporate a variety of exercises that target all aspects of the core for a well-rounded workout routine.

- **Myth #2:** You need fancy equipment to strengthen your core. While fancy equipment like stability balls, resistance bands, and ab machines can add variety to your workouts, they're by no means necessary for building a strong core. In fact, many effective core exercises can be performed using nothing more than your body weight and a mat. Planks, mountain climbers, and bicycle crunches are just a few examples of equipment-free exercises that can challenge your core muscles and deliver results.

- **Myth #3:** Core strength is all about aesthetics. While having a toned, defined midsection may be a desirable side effect of core training, the true purpose of core strength goes far beyond mere aesthetics. A strong core is essential for maintaining spinal health, preventing injury, and enhancing overall functional performance. Whether you're an athlete looking to improve your athletic performance or an everyday individual striving to move with ease and confidence, core strength is a cornerstone of physical fitness that should not be overlooked.

By dispelling these common myths and gaining a deeper understanding of core anatomy and functionality, you'll be better equipped to embark on a core exercise journey that is both effective and sustainable. So, bid farewell to misconceptions, embrace the complexity of your core, and get ready to unleash your full potential. The journey to a stronger, more resilient core begins with knowledge, dedication, and a willingness to challenge the status quo.

ESSENTIAL CORE EXERCISES

Welcome to the heart of your core workout journey! In this chapter, we'll explore a variety of essential core exercises designed to target different aspects of your core musculature. From mastering proper form and technique to diving into specific exercises, get ready to feel the burn and unleash your core strength.

Proper Form and Technique Guidelines

Before we dive into the specific exercises, let's talk about the importance of proper form and technique when it comes to core training. Proper form not only maximizes the effectiveness of each exercise but also reduces the risk of injury and ensures that you're targeting the intended muscle groups.

First and foremost, focus on maintaining a neutral spine throughout each exercise. This means keeping your spine in a natural alignment, with your head, neck, and spine forming a straight line. Avoid overarching or rounding your back, as this can put undue stress on the spine and increase the risk of injury.

Next, engage your core muscles throughout each movement. Imagine drawing your belly button in towards your spine to activate the deep stabilizing muscles of the core, such as the transverse abdominis. This helps to create stability and support for your spine, allowing you to perform the exercises with control and precision.

Additionally, pay attention to your breathing pattern. Inhale deeply through your nose during the eccentric (lowering) phase of the exercise, and exhale forcefully through your mouth during the concentric (lifting) phase. This rhythmic breathing helps to oxygenate your muscles and maintain proper intra-abdominal pressure.

Lastly, start with a light warm-up to prepare your body for the upcoming workout. This could include dynamic movements such as arm circles, leg swings, and torso twists to increase blood flow to the muscles and loosen up tight areas.

By focusing on proper form and technique, you'll not only maximize the benefits of each exercise but also reduce the risk of injury and ensure a safe and effective workout.

5-Minute Plank Variations

Ah, the plank a classic core exercise that never fails to challenge even the fittest of individuals. But did you know that there are countless variations to this staple exercise? Let's explore a few plank variations that will test your core strength and endurance in new and exciting ways.

- **Standard Plank**: Begin in a push-up position with your hands directly beneath your shoulders and your body forming a straight line from head to heels. Engage your core muscles and hold this position for as long as possible, aiming for at least 30 seconds to start.
- **Side Plank**: Lie on your side with your legs stacked and your elbow directly beneath your shoulder. Lift your hips off the ground, creating a straight line from head to heels. Hold this position, engaging your oblique's and maintaining stability throughout your core.

- **Plank with Leg Lifts**: From a standard plank position, lift one leg off the ground, keeping it straight and parallel to the floor. Hold for a few seconds before returning to the starting position. Repeat on the other side, alternating legs for the duration of the exercise.

- **Plank with Shoulder Taps**: In a standard plank position, lift one hand off the ground and tap the opposite shoulder. Return to the starting position and repeat on the other side, alternating sides for the duration of the exercise. Focus on maintaining stability through your core and minimizing hip rotation.

- **Plank Jacks**: Begin in a standard plank position. Jump your feet out wide, then back together, keeping your core engaged and your hips stable. Continue to alternate between jumping your feet in and out for the duration of the exercise, maintaining a steady pace and focusing on control.

Incorporate these plank variations into your core workout routine to add variety and challenge your muscles in new ways. Remember to maintain proper form and technique throughout each exercise, and listen to your body to avoid overexertion or injury.

Crunches: Variations and Modifications

Ah, the humble crunch a timeless staple of core training. While traditional crunches are effective for targeting the rectus abdominis, there are countless variations and modifications to spice up your core workout routine. Let's explore a few options to keep your abs engaged and your workouts interesting.

- **Basic Crunch**: Lie on your back with your knees bent and feet flat on the floor. Place your hands behind your head or across your chest. Engage your core and lift your shoulders off the ground, curling towards your knees. Lower back down with control, keeping your lower back pressed into the mat.

- **Reverse Crunch**: Begin lying on your back with your arms by your sides and your legs lifted towards the ceiling, knees bent at a 90-degree angle. Engage your core and lift your hips off the ground, bringing your knees towards your chest. Lower back down with control, maintaining stability through your core.

- **Bicycle Crunches**: Lie on your back with your knees bent and hands behind your head. Lift your shoulders off the ground and bring your right elbow towards your left knee, simultaneously extending your right leg out straight. Repeat on the other side, alternating between left and right for the duration of the exercise.

- **Toe Touch Crunches**: Lie on your back with your legs extended towards the ceiling and your arms reaching towards your toes. Engage your core and lift your shoulders off the ground, reaching your hands towards your toes. Lower back down with control, focusing on the contraction of your abdominal muscles.

- **Oblique Crunches**: Lie on your back with your knees bent and feet flat on the floor. Place your hands behind your head and cross your left ankle over your right knee. Engage your core and lift your shoulders off the ground, rotating towards your left knee. Lower back down with control and repeat on the other side.

Incorporate these crunch variations into your core workout routine to target different areas of your abdominals and keep your muscles guessing. Remember to focus on quality over quantity, maintaining proper form and technique throughout each repetition.

Russian Twists: A Dynamic Core Exercise

Ready to add a twist literally to your core workout routine? Enter the Russian twist, a dynamic exercise that targets your oblique's, transverse abdominis, and hip flexors with every rotation. Let's break down the proper form and technique for this challenging yet rewarding exercise.

- **Basic Russian Twist**: Sit on the ground with your knees bent and feet flat on the floor, hip-width apart. Lean back slightly, engaging your core to maintain a straight spine. Clasp your hands together in front of your chest or hold a weight for added resistance.

- **Twisting Motion**: From the starting position, engage your core and twist your torso to the right, bringing your hands or weight towards the ground outside of your right hip. Keep your chest lifted and your spine tall throughout the movement.

- **Return to Center**: Reverse the twisting motion, bringing your hands or weight back to the center of your body. Pause briefly before twisting to the left, bringing your hands or weight towards the ground outside of your left hip.

- **Repeat**: Continue to alternate between twisting to the right and left, maintaining a controlled and steady pace. Focus on engaging your oblique's and avoiding excessive movement in your hips or shoulders.

- **Advanced Variation**: To increase the intensity of the exercise, lift your feet off the ground and balance on your sit bones. This challenges your core stability and adds an extra element of difficulty to the exercise.

Incorporate Russian twists into your core workout routine to target your oblique's and improve rotational strength and stability. Start with a light weight or no weight at all, focusing on proper form and technique before progressing to heavier resistance.

Superman Pose: Strengthening Your Lower Back

While many core exercises focus on the abdominals, it's essential not to neglect the muscles of the lower back. The Superman pose is a simple yet effective exercise that targets the erector spinae and other muscles of the lower back, helping to improve spinal stability and posture.

- **Starting Position**: Begin lying face down on the ground with your arms extended overhead and your legs straight behind you. Engage your core and glutes to support your spine and maintain a neutral position.

- **Lift Upper Body**: Inhale deeply and lift your chest, arms, and legs off the ground simultaneously. Keep your gaze forward and your neck in a neutral position to avoid straining your cervical spine.

- **Hold and Squeeze**: Hold the lifted position for a few seconds, focusing on squeezing your glutes and engaging your lower back muscles. Imagine lengthening through your fingertips and toes to create a straight line from head to heels.

- **Lower with Control**: Exhale slowly as you lower your chest, arms, and legs back to the starting position. Maintain control throughout the movement, avoiding any sudden or jerky motions.

- **Repeat**: Perform several repetitions of the Superman pose, aiming for 10-15 reps per set. Focus on maintaining proper form and technique, and listen to your body to avoid overexertion or strain.

Incorporate the Superman pose into your core workout routine to strengthen the muscles of your lower back and improve overall spinal stability. Remember to start with a light lift and gradually increase the intensity as you build strength and confidence in the exercise.

Bicycle Crunches: Engaging Your Entire Core

Looking for a challenging core exercise that targets multiple muscle groups simultaneously? Enter the bicycle crunch a dynamic movement that engages your entire core, including the rectus abdominis, oblique's, and hip flexors. Let's dive into the proper form and technique for mastering this powerhouse exercise.

- **Starting Position**: Lie on your back with your knees bent and feet flat on the floor. Place your hands behind your head, elbows pointing out to the sides, and lift your shoulders off the ground to engage your core.

- **Bicycle Motion**: Begin by bringing your right knee towards your chest while simultaneously rotating your torso to bring your left elbow towards your right knee. Imagine pedaling a bicycle as you extend your left leg out straight.

- **Alternate Sides**: Reverse the motion, bringing your left knee towards your chest while rotating your torso to bring your right elbow towards your left knee. Continue to alternate between left and right, mimicking the motion of pedaling a bicycle.

- **Focus on Control**: Maintain a steady and controlled pace throughout the exercise, focusing on the contraction of your abdominal muscles with each repetition. Avoid rushing through the movement or using momentum to swing your legs.

- **Breathe**: Remember to breathe rhythmically throughout the exercise, inhaling deeply as you rotate and exhaling as you return to the starting position. This helps to oxygenate your muscles and maintain proper intra-abdominal pressure.

Incorporate bicycle crunches into your core workout routine to target your entire core and improve strength, endurance, and stability. Start with a few sets of 10-15 reps, gradually increasing the intensity and duration as you build strength and confidence in the exercise.

Mountain Climbers: Cardio and Core Combination

Looking for a core exercise that doubles as a cardio workout? Look no further than mountain climbers—a dynamic movement that targets your core, shoulders, and legs while also elevating your heart rate for a calorie-burning cardio blast. Let's explore how to perform mountain climbers with proper form and technique.

- **Starting Position**: Begin in a high plank position with your hands directly beneath your shoulders and your body forming a straight line from head to heels. Engage your core and glutes to maintain stability throughout your body.

- **Driving Motion**: Start by bringing your right knee towards your chest, keeping your foot off the ground. Engage your core and drive your knee forward with power and control.

- **Switching Legs**: As you return your right foot to the starting position, immediately drive your left knee towards your chest in a smooth and fluid motion. Alternate between left and right, mimicking the motion of running in place.

- **Maintain Tempo**: Aim for a steady and controlled pace throughout the exercise, moving as quickly as you can while maintaining proper form and technique. Focus on engaging your core and minimizing any rocking or swaying of your hips.

- **Breathe**: Remember to breathe rhythmically throughout the exercise, inhaling and exhaling with each repetition. This helps to oxygenate your muscles and maintain a steady flow of energy throughout your body.

Incorporate mountain climbers into your core workout routine to add a cardio component and elevate your heart rate for a calorie-burning, full-body workout. Start with 30-second intervals, gradually increasing the duration as you build strength and endurance.

By incorporating these essential core exercises into your workout routine, you'll target all aspects of your core musculature and build strength, stability, and endurance from the inside out. Remember to focus on proper form and technique, listen to your body, and progress at your own pace. With dedication, consistency, and a bit of sweat, you'll be well on your way to achieving your core fitness goals.

THE BENEFITS OF CORE EXERCISE

Core exercise goes beyond just achieving a six-pack; it's about cultivating strength, stability, and resilience throughout your entire body. In this chapter, we'll explore the myriad benefits of core exercise, including improving posture and balance, enhancing athletic performance, reducing the risk of injury, and boosting functional fitness.

Improving Posture and Balance

One of the most significant benefits of core exercise is its positive impact on posture and balance. Your core muscles, which include not only your abdominals but also your lower back, hips, and pelvis, play a crucial role in maintaining proper alignment and stability throughout your body.

When your core muscles are weak or imbalanced, it can lead to poor posture, which can contribute to a range of musculoskeletal issues, including back pain, neck pain, and joint discomfort. By strengthening and stabilizing your core muscles, you can improve your posture and reduce the risk of developing these common ailments.

Core exercises such as planks, bird dogs, and bridges target the deep muscles of the abdomen, lower back, and pelvis, helping to improve core strength, stability, and alignment. These exercises encourage proper spinal alignment and pelvic positioning, which can translate to better posture both during exercise and in everyday activities.

In addition to improving posture, core exercise also enhances balance and coordination, which are essential for preventing falls and maintaining mobility as you age. By challenging your core muscles in various planes of motion and incorporating dynamic movements into your workouts, you can improve your body's ability to maintain stability and balance, reducing the risk of falls and injuries.

Enhancing Athletic Performance

Core strength and stability are fundamental components of athletic performance across a wide range of sports and activities. Whether you're a competitive athlete or a recreational fitness enthusiast, a strong and stable core can help improve your performance and prevent injuries.

In sports that require explosive power and agility, such as basketball, soccer, and tennis, a strong core is essential for generating power, transferring force, and maintaining balance and control during rapid movements. By incorporating core exercises into your training routine, you can enhance your ability to accelerate, decelerate, change direction, and perform explosive movements with greater efficiency and precision.

In addition to power and agility, core strength also plays a critical role in endurance sports such as running, cycling, and swimming. A strong core helps maintain proper posture and alignment, reducing fatigue and inefficiency over long distances. By improving core strength and stability, you can optimize your biomechanics and energy efficiency, allowing you to perform at your best for longer periods without succumbing to fatigue or injury.

Reducing Risk of Injury

Weak or imbalanced core muscles can increase the risk of injury, both during exercise and in everyday activities. When your core muscles are unable to provide adequate support and stability, it can lead to compensatory movement patterns, muscle imbalances, and overuse injuries in other areas of the body.

By incorporating core exercises into your training routine, you can strengthen and stabilize the muscles surrounding your spine, pelvis, and hips, reducing the risk of injury and improving overall movement quality and efficiency. Strong core muscles act as a protective shield for your spine and joints, helping to absorb shock and distribute forces more evenly throughout your body, reducing the risk of strain, sprain, or overuse injuries.

In addition to preventing injuries, core exercise can also help rehabilitate and recover from existing injuries by improving muscle strength, flexibility, and stability. Exercises such as plank variations, bird dogs, and bridges can be particularly beneficial for individuals recovering from back pain, hip pain, or other musculoskeletal injuries, as they target the deep stabilizing muscles of the core without placing excessive stress on the joints.

Boosting Functional Fitness

Functional fitness refers to the ability to perform everyday activities with ease and efficiency, without undue strain or discomfort. A strong and stable core is essential for supporting functional movements such as bending, twisting, lifting, and reaching, which are required for tasks ranging from household chores to recreational activities to work-related tasks.

By incorporating core exercises into your training routine, you can improve your body's ability to perform these functional movements safely and effectively, reducing the risk of injury and enhancing your overall quality of life. Core exercises such as squats, lunges, and deadlifts mimic the movements of everyday activities, helping to strengthen the muscles involved in bending, lifting, and carrying objects. In addition to supporting functional movements, core exercise can also improve your body's overall resilience and durability, allowing you to withstand the physical demands of daily life with greater ease and confidence. Whether you're picking up groceries, playing with your kids, or participating in recreational sports, a strong and stable core will help you move more efficiently, reduce the risk of injury, and enjoy life to the fullest.

core exercise offers a wide range of benefits that extend far beyond aesthetics. By improving posture and balance, enhancing athletic performance, reducing the risk of injury, and boosting functional fitness, core exercise plays a crucial role in promoting overall health, well-being, and quality of life. Whether you're an athlete looking to improve performance, an active individual seeking to prevent injuries, or someone simply looking to feel stronger and more confident in your daily activities, incorporating core exercises into your training routine can help you achieve your goals and live life to the fullest.

ADVANCED CORE CHALLENGES

Congratulations on reaching the advanced level of your core training journey! As you continue to build strength, stability, and endurance, it's time to take your workouts to the next level with a variety of challenging exercises and techniques. In this chapter, we'll explore advanced core challenges designed to push your limits and unlock new levels of strength and performance.

Graduating from Beginner to Intermediate Level

Before we delve into the advanced exercises, let's take a moment to acknowledge how far you've come since starting your core training journey. By mastering the basics and building a solid foundation of strength and stability, you've laid the groundwork for continued progress and success.

As you transition from beginner to intermediate level, you'll notice improvements in your core strength, endurance, and overall fitness. Movements that once felt challenging will become more manageable, and you'll have the confidence to tackle new challenges with ease.

But don't get too comfortable just yet there's still plenty of room for growth and improvement. By embracing the mindset of continual progression and pushing yourself outside your comfort zone, you'll continue to see gains in strength, performance, and physique.

Increasing Intensity Safely

As you advance in your core training journey, it's important to increase the intensity of your workouts gradually and safely. Rapidly ramping up the intensity can lead to overtraining, burnout, and increased risk of injury, so it's crucial to proceed with caution and listen to your body.

One way to increase intensity safely is to gradually increase the duration or intensity of your workouts over time. For example, you might add an extra set of repetitions to each exercise or increase the resistance or difficulty level of certain movements.

Another strategy is to incorporate interval training into your workouts, alternating between periods of high-intensity exercise and recovery. This not only challenges your cardiovascular system but also helps to boost calorie burn and accelerate fat loss.

Additionally, be sure to incorporate adequate rest and recovery into your routine to allow your muscles time to repair and rebuild. Overtraining can lead to diminished performance, increased risk of injury, and burnout, so it's essential to strike a balance between challenging yourself and giving your body the rest it needs to thrive.

By increasing intensity safely and gradually, you'll continue to see progress and improvements in your core strength, endurance, and overall fitness without compromising your health or well-being.

Incorporating Equipment: Stability Ball, Resistance Bands, etc.

Ready to kick your core workouts up a notch? Incorporating equipment such as stability balls, resistance bands, and medicine balls can add variety, challenge, and fun to your workouts while targeting different muscle groups and movement patterns.

- **Stability Ball**: Incorporating a stability ball into your core workouts adds an element of instability, forcing your core muscles to work harder to maintain balance and control. Exercises such as stability ball crunches, pikes, and rollouts target the abdominals, obliques, and lower back while also engaging stabilizing muscles throughout the body.

- **Resistance Bands**: Resistance bands are versatile tools that can be used to add resistance to traditional core exercises or to target specific muscle groups with isolation movements. Try incorporating resistance band crunches, side bends, and seated twists into your routine to challenge your core muscles from different angles and planes of motion.

- **Medicine Ball**: Medicine balls are excellent for adding resistance and dynamic movement to your core workouts. Exercises such as medicine ball slams, twists, and Russian twists engage the core muscles while also improving coordination, power, and explosiveness.

- **TRX Suspension Trainer**: The TRX suspension trainer is a portable training tool that uses your body weight and gravity to create resistance. Suspended core exercises such as TRX planks, pikes, and knee tucks challenge your core stability and strength while also engaging other muscles throughout the body.

Incorporating equipment into your core workouts adds variety, challenge, and excitement while targeting different muscle groups and movement patterns. Experiment with different tools and exercises to find what works best for you and keep your workouts fresh and engaging.

Advanced Plank Variations

Ready to take your plank game to the next level? Advanced plank variations add an extra challenge to this classic core exercise, targeting different muscle groups and movement patterns while building strength, stability, and endurance.

- **Plank with Knee Tucks**: Start in a high plank position with your hands directly beneath your shoulders and your body forming a straight line from head to heels. Engage your core and lift your hips towards the ceiling, bringing your knees towards your chest in a controlled manner. Return to the starting position and repeat for the desired number of repetitions.

- **Side Plank with Hip Dips**: Begin in a side plank position with your elbow directly beneath your shoulder and your body forming a straight line from head to heels. Engage your core and lower your hips towards the ground, then lift them back up to the starting position. Repeat on the other side, alternating between left and right for the desired number of repetitions.

- **Plank with Shoulder Taps and Leg Lifts**: Start in a high plank position with your hands directly beneath your shoulders and your body forming a straight line from head to heels. Engage your core and lift one hand off the ground to tap the opposite shoulder, then lift the opposite leg off the ground to hip height. Return to the starting position and repeat on the other side, alternating between left and right for the desired number of repetitions.

- **Plank with Alternating Arm and Leg Lifts**: Begin in a high plank position with your hands directly beneath your shoulders and your body forming a straight line from head to heels. Engage your core and lift one arm and the opposite leg off the ground simultaneously, extending them out straight. Return to the starting position and repeat on the other side, alternating between left and right for the desired number of repetitions.

- **Plank with Spider-Man Crunches**: Start in a high plank position with your hands directly beneath your shoulders and your body forming a straight line from head to heels. Engage your core and bring your right knee towards your right elbow in a controlled manner, then return to the starting position and repeat on the other side, alternating between left and right for the desired number of repetitions.

Incorporate these advanced plank variations into your core workout routine to add variety, challenge, and excitement while targeting different muscle groups and movement patterns. Remember to focus on proper form and technique, and listen to your body to avoid overexertion or injury.

V-Ups: Taking Your Core Work to the Next Level

Ready to challenge your core with an advanced exercise that targets your abdominals, hip flexors, and lower back? Enter the V-up an intense movement that requires strength, stability, and coordination to perform correctly.

- **Starting Position**: Lie on your back with your arms extended overhead and your legs straight out in front of you. Engage your core and lift your upper body and legs off the ground simultaneously, forming a V shape with your body.

- **Upward Motion**: Reach towards your toes with your hands while simultaneously lifting your legs towards the ceiling. Keep your core engaged and your spine straight throughout the movement, avoiding any arching or rounding of the back.

- **Balancing Act**: Hold the lifted position for a moment, focusing on maintaining stability and control. Imagine lengthening through your fingertips and toes to create a long, straight line from head to heels.

- **Lowering with Control**: Slowly lower your upper body and legs back to the starting position, maintaining tension in your core muscles throughout the descent. Avoid letting your shoulders or feet touch the ground until you've completed the desired number of repetitions.

- **Repeat**: Perform several repetitions of the V-up, aiming for 8-12 reps per set. Focus on quality over quantity, and listen to your body to avoid overexertion or strain.

Incorporate V-ups into your core workout routine to challenge your abdominal muscles, improve core strength and stability, and take your core training to the next level. Start with a few sets of moderate reps, gradually increasing the intensity and duration as you build strength and confidence in the exercise.

Leg Raises: Building Lower Abdominal Strength

Looking to target your lower abs and build strength and definition in your lower abdominal region? Leg raises are an effective exercise that isolates the muscles of the lower abs while also engaging the hip flexors and lower back.

- **Starting Position**: Lie on your back with your legs extended and your arms by your sides. Engage your core and lift your legs off the ground, keeping them straight and together.

- **Upward Motion**: Slowly raise your legs towards the ceiling, lifting your hips off the ground as high as you can without arching your lower back. Focus on using your lower abs to initiate the movement, rather than relying on momentum or swinging your legs.

- **Controlled Descent**: Lower your legs back down to the starting position with control, avoiding any sudden or jerky movements. Keep tension in your core muscles throughout the descent to maximize the effectiveness of the exercise.

- **Breathing**: Remember to breathe rhythmically throughout the exercise, inhaling as you raise your legs and exhaling as you lower them back down. This helps to oxygenate your muscles and maintain proper intra-abdominal pressure.

- **Repeat**: Perform several repetitions of leg raises, aiming for 10-15 reps per set. Focus on maintaining proper form and technique, and listen to your body to avoid overexertion or strain.

Incorporate leg raises into your core workout routine to target your lower abs, improve core strength and stability, and enhance overall muscle definition in your abdominal region. Start with a few sets of moderate reps, gradually increasing the intensity and duration as you build strength and confidence in the exercise.

These advanced core challenges into your workout routine, you'll continue to push your limits, unlock new levels of strength and performance, and achieve your fitness goals. Remember to focus on proper form and technique, listen to your body, and progress at your own pace. With dedication, consistency, and a willingness to step outside your comfort zone, you'll continue to see progress and improvements in your core strength, endurance, and overall fitness.

CRAFTING YOUR CORE WORKOUT ROUTINE

Congratulations on reaching the stage where you're ready to craft a core workout routine that suits your needs and helps you achieve your fitness goals. In this chapter, we'll explore the essential components of designing an effective core workout plan, incorporating rest days and recovery, tracking your progress, and dealing with plateaus and challenges along the way.

Designing a Balanced Workout Plan

When it comes to crafting a core workout routine, balance is key. A well-rounded plan should include a mix of exercises that target all areas of the core, including the rectus abdominis, oblique's, transverse abdominis, and lower back muscles. Additionally, it's essential to incorporate variety into your routine to prevent boredom, challenge your muscles in new ways, and avoid overuse injuries.

Begin by selecting a variety of exercises that target different aspects of the core musculature. This could include exercises such as planks, crunches, Russian twists, leg raises, and stability ball exercises. Aim to include exercises that target both the front and sides of the core, as well as exercises that focus on stability and balance.

Next, consider the intensity and volume of your workouts. Gradually increase the difficulty of your exercises over time by adding resistance, increasing repetitions, or incorporating more challenging variations. However, be mindful not to push yourself too hard, especially if you're new to core training or recovering from an injury. Listen to your body and adjust the intensity of your workouts as needed.

Finally, don't forget to include rest days in your workout plan. Rest days are crucial for allowing your muscles to repair and rebuild, reducing the risk of overtraining and burnout. Aim to include at least one or two rest days per week, during which you can engage in light activity such as walking, yoga, or stretching to promote recovery and relaxation.

By designing a balanced workout plan that includes a variety of exercises targeting all aspects of the core, gradually increasing the intensity and volume of your workouts over time, and incorporating rest days for recovery, you'll set yourself up for success in achieving your fitness goals.

Incorporating Rest Days and Recovery

Rest days are just as important as your workout days when it comes to achieving your fitness goals. They allow your muscles time to repair and rebuild, reduce the risk of overtraining and injury, and help prevent burnout. However, rest days don't necessarily mean lounging on the couch all day—they can also include light activity such as walking, yoga, or stretching to promote recovery and relaxation.

When incorporating rest days into your workout routine, aim to include at least one or two days per week where you engage in minimal or no intense exercise. Listen to your body and pay attention to signs of fatigue, soreness, or decreased performance, which may indicate that you need to take an extra rest day.

Additionally, prioritize recovery strategies such as proper nutrition, hydration, and sleep to support your body's recovery process. Ensure that you're consuming an adequate amount of protein, carbohydrates, and healthy fats to fuel your muscles and promote muscle repair and growth. Stay hydrated by drinking plenty of water throughout the day, and aim for 7-9 hours of quality sleep each night to allow your body to rest and rejuvenate.

Incorporating rest days and prioritizing recovery strategies into your workout routine is essential for maintaining optimal performance, preventing injury, and achieving your fitness goals in the long term. Remember that rest is not a sign of weakness—it's an essential component of a balanced and sustainable approach to fitness.

Tracking Your Progress

Tracking your progress is an essential aspect of any fitness journey, providing valuable insight into your strengths, weaknesses, and areas for improvement. By monitoring key metrics such as strength, endurance, and body composition, you can assess your progress over time and make informed decisions about your training program.

One of the most straightforward ways to track your progress is by keeping a workout journal or log. Record details such as the exercises you performed, the number of sets and repetitions, the amount of weight lifted, and any notes about your performance or how you felt during the workout. This allows you to track your progress over time and identify trends or patterns in your training.

Additionally, consider incorporating measurements such as body weight, body fat percentage, and circumference measurements into your tracking routine. While these metrics don't tell the whole story, they can provide valuable insight into changes in your body composition and overall progress towards your goals.

Another useful tool for tracking progress is keeping a visual record of your workouts. Take photos or videos of yourself performing exercises at regular intervals to visually track changes in your physique, posture, and movement patterns over time. This can be especially helpful for identifying areas of improvement and celebrating milestones along the way.

Finally, don't forget to celebrate your progress and achievements along the way. Whether it's hitting a new personal best in the gym, achieving a milestone in your body composition goals, or mastering a challenging exercise, take the time to acknowledge and celebrate your successes. This not only boosts your confidence and motivation but also reinforces positive behaviors and habits that contribute to long-term success.

By tracking your progress regularly and consistently, you'll gain valuable insights into your training program, identify areas for improvement, and stay motivated and focused on your fitness goals.

Dealing with Plateaus and Challenges

Plateaus and challenges are an inevitable part of any fitness journey, but they don't have to derail your progress or dampen your motivation. By understanding the common causes of plateaus and challenges and implementing strategies to overcome them, you can continue making progress towards your goals and achieve long-term success.

One common cause of plateaus is sticking to the same routine for too long without making any changes. Your body adapts to the demands placed on it, so it's essential to periodically change up your workouts to continue challenging your muscles and stimulating growth. Incorporate new exercises, vary the intensity and volume of your workouts, or try different training modalities such as HIIT or circuit training to keep your body guessing and prevent plateaus.

Another common cause of plateaus is improper nutrition or hydration. Ensure that you're fueling your body with the nutrients it needs to support your workouts and recovery, including an adequate amount of protein, carbohydrates, and healthy fats. Stay hydrated by drinking plenty of water throughout the day, as dehydration can negatively impact performance and recovery.

Additionally, be mindful of external factors that may affect your progress, such as stress, sleep, and lifestyle habits. Chronic stress can elevate cortisol levels, which can interfere with muscle growth and recovery. Aim to manage stress through relaxation techniques such as meditation, deep breathing, or yoga, and prioritize quality sleep to allow your body to rest and recover fully.

Finally, don't be afraid to seek support and guidance from a qualified fitness professional if you're struggling to overcome a plateau or facing challenges in your training. A personal trainer or coach can provide personalized advice, guidance, and accountability to help you break through barriers, overcome obstacles, and achieve your fitness goals.

By understanding the common causes of plateaus and challenges, implementing strategies to overcome them, and seeking support when needed, you can continue making progress towards your goals and achieve long-term success in your fitness journey. Remember that progress takes time, consistency, and patience, so stay focused, stay motivated, and keep pushing forward towards your goals.

Crafting your core workout routine is an exciting and empowering process that allows you to tailor your workouts to your unique needs and goals. By designing a balanced workout plan, incorporating rest days and recovery, tracking your progress, and dealing with plateaus and challenges along the way, you'll set yourself up for success in achieving your fitness goals and living a healthy, active lifestyle.

NUTRITION AND CORE STRENGTH

Nutrition plays a fundamental role in all aspects of health and fitness, including core strength and development. In this chapter, we'll explore the importance of nutrition in core development, discuss foods that support muscle growth and recovery, and delve into the essential role of hydration in maintaining a strong core.

The Role of Nutrition in Core Development

When it comes to building a strong and resilient core, nutrition is just as important as exercise. Your core muscles require adequate nutrients to repair and rebuild after workouts, support muscle growth, and maintain optimal function. Additionally, proper nutrition can help reduce inflammation, improve energy levels, and support overall health and well-being.

One essential nutrient for core development is protein. Protein is the building block of muscle tissue and is crucial for repairing and rebuilding muscles after exercise. Aim to include a source of protein in each meal and snack throughout the day, such as lean meats, poultry, fish, eggs, dairy products, legumes, tofu, and tempeh.

In addition to protein, carbohydrates are an important source of energy for your workouts and support recovery by replenishing glycogen stores in your muscles. Choose complex carbohydrates such as whole grains, fruits, vegetables, and legumes, which provide sustained energy and essential nutrients.

Healthy fats are also important for overall health and can support core development by reducing inflammation and providing sustained energy.

Incorporate sources of healthy fats such as avocados, nuts, seeds, olive oil, and fatty fish into your diet to support your core training efforts.

Lastly, don't forget about micronutrients such as vitamins and minerals, which play a vital role in muscle function, energy production, and overall health. Aim to eat a varied and balanced diet rich in fruits, vegetables, whole grains, and lean proteins to ensure you're getting a wide range of essential nutrients to support your core development.

By fueling your body with a balanced diet rich in protein, carbohydrates, healthy fats, and essential nutrients, you'll provide your core muscles with the fuel they need to thrive, support muscle growth and recovery, and optimize your performance in the gym and beyond.

Foods That Support Muscle Growth and Recovery

In addition to providing your body with essential nutrients, certain foods can specifically support muscle growth and recovery, making them valuable additions to your diet as you work to develop a strong and resilient core.

One of the most important nutrients for muscle growth and recovery is protein. Protein provides the building blocks your muscles need to repair and rebuild after exercise, supporting muscle growth and strength. Opt for high-quality sources of protein such as lean meats, poultry, fish, eggs, dairy products, legumes, and plant-based protein sources such as tofu and tempeh.

In addition to protein, foods rich in complex carbohydrates can provide the energy your muscles need to fuel intense workouts and support recovery afterward. Choose whole grains such as brown rice, quinoa, oats, and barley, as well as fruits, vegetables, and legumes, which provide a steady source of energy and essential nutrients.

Healthy fats are also important for muscle growth and recovery, as they provide sustained energy and support overall health and well-being. Incorporate sources of healthy fats such as avocados, nuts, seeds, olive oil, and fatty fish into your diet to support your core training efforts.

Lastly, don't forget about hydration. Proper hydration is essential for muscle function, recovery, and overall performance. Aim to drink plenty of water throughout the day, especially before, during, and after exercise, to stay hydrated and support optimal muscle function and recovery.

By incorporating these foods into your diet regularly, you'll provide your body with the nutrients it needs to support muscle growth and recovery, optimize your performance in the gym, and achieve your core strength and fitness goals.

Hydration: Why It's Essential for a Strong Core

Hydration plays a crucial role in all aspects of health and fitness, including core strength and development. Proper hydration is essential for maintaining optimal muscle function, supporting energy production, and facilitating recovery after exercise.

Water makes up a significant portion of your muscle tissue, and dehydration can impair muscle function and performance. When you're dehydrated, your muscles may feel fatigued, cramp more easily, and take longer to recover after exercise. Proper hydration ensures that your muscles are functioning optimally, allowing you to perform at your best during workouts and recover more quickly afterward.

In addition to supporting muscle function and recovery, hydration is also essential for maintaining optimal energy levels during exercise. Dehydration can lead to fatigue, decreased endurance, and diminished performance, making it harder to complete your workouts with intensity and focus. By staying properly hydrated, you'll ensure that your body has the energy it needs to power through your workouts and achieve your fitness goals.

Proper hydration is also crucial for supporting overall health and well-being. Water plays a vital role in regulating body temperature, aiding digestion, transporting nutrients, and removing waste products from the body. Dehydration can impair these essential functions, leading to a range of health issues and symptoms such as headaches, dizziness, and decreased cognitive function.

To stay properly hydrated, aim to drink plenty of water throughout the day, especially before, during, and after exercise. The exact amount of water you need will depend on factors such as your body size, activity level, and environmental conditions, but a good rule of thumb is to aim for at least 8-10 cups of water per day, or more if you're active or exercising in hot weather.

In addition to water, you can also stay hydrated by consuming hydrating foods such as fruits and vegetables, which have high water content and provide additional nutrients and electrolytes to support hydration and overall health.

By prioritizing hydration and ensuring that you're properly hydrated before, during, and after exercise, you'll support optimal muscle function, energy production, and recovery, allowing you to perform at your best and achieve your core strength and fitness goals.

nutrition plays a critical role in core strength and development, providing the essential nutrients your muscles need to repair, rebuild, and grow stronger. By fueling your body with a balanced diet rich in protein, carbohydrates, healthy fats, and essential nutrients, you'll provide your core muscles with the fuel they need to thrive and support optimal performance in the gym and beyond. Additionally, proper hydration is essential for maintaining optimal muscle function, supporting energy production, and facilitating recovery after exercise. By staying properly hydrated and prioritizing hydration before, during, and after exercise, you'll support optimal muscle function, energy production, and recovery, allowing you to perform at your best and achieve your core strength and fitness goals.

AVOIDING COMMON MISTAKES

In your journey to develop a strong and functional core, it's important to be aware of common mistakes that can hinder your progress and even lead to injury. In this chapter, we'll explore some of these pitfalls and provide guidance on how to avoid them, focusing on overtraining and injury prevention, listening to your body, and balancing core work with other fitness activities.

Overtraining and Injury Prevention

One of the most common mistakes people make when it comes to core training is overdoing it. While it's important to challenge your muscles and push yourself outside your comfort zone, overtraining can lead to burnout, fatigue, and increased risk of injury. Here are some tips to help you avoid overtraining and stay injury-free:

- **Progress Gradually**: When starting a new core training program, it can be tempting to dive in headfirst and push yourself to the limit. However, this approach can increase the risk of injury and burnout. Instead, progress gradually, starting with lighter weights and fewer repetitions and gradually increasing the intensity and volume of your workouts over time.

- **Listen to Your Body**: Pay attention to how your body feels during and after your workouts. If you experience persistent pain, discomfort, or fatigue, it may be a sign that you're pushing yourself too hard and need to dial back the intensity or take a rest day. Ignoring these warning signs can lead to overuse injuries and setbacks in your training.

- **Include Rest Days**: Rest days are essential for allowing your muscles time to repair and recover after intense workouts. Aim to include at least one or two rest days per week, during which you engage in light activity such as walking, yoga, or stretching to promote recovery and relaxation. This will help prevent overtraining and keep you feeling fresh and energized for your next workout.

- **Cross-Train**: In addition to core-specific exercises, incorporate a variety of activities into your fitness routine to prevent overuse injuries and promote overall strength and fitness. Include activities such as strength training, cardiovascular exercise, flexibility training, and mobility work to ensure a well-rounded approach to fitness and reduce the risk of overtraining specific muscle groups.

By following these tips and being mindful of your body's signals, you can avoid overtraining and reduce the risk of injury, allowing you to progress safely and effectively in your core training journey.

Listening to Your Body

Listening to your body is perhaps one of the most important principles to abide by in any fitness endeavor, including core training. Your body is incredibly intelligent and will often provide signals and feedback that can guide your training and help you avoid injury. Here's how to tune in and listen to what your body is telling you:

- **Pay Attention to Pain**: Pain is your body's way of signaling that something is wrong. While some discomfort during workouts is normal, persistent or sharp pain could indicate an injury or overuse issue. If you experience pain, stop the exercise immediately and assess the situation. Ignoring pain and pushing through can lead to further injury and setbacks in your training.

- **Respect Fatigue**: Feeling tired or fatigued during or after a workout is normal, especially if you're pushing yourself to improve. However, it's essential to distinguish between normal fatigue and excessive exhaustion. If you consistently feel drained or depleted, it may be a sign that you're overtraining and need to scale back your workouts or incorporate more rest days into your routine.

- **Listen to Your Instincts**: Trust your intuition and listen to what your body is telling you. If something doesn't feel right or if a particular exercise doesn't agree with your body, don't force it. There are plenty of ways to work your core muscles effectively without causing discomfort or pain. Experiment with different exercises and variations to find what works best for you and your body.

- **Prioritize Recovery**: Recovery is just as important as the workout itself when it comes to achieving your fitness goals. Make sure you're giving your body the rest and recovery it needs to repair and rebuild after intense workouts. This includes getting enough sleep, staying hydrated, eating a balanced diet, and incorporating rest days into your routine.

By tuning in and listening to your body's signals, you can avoid injury, prevent overtraining, and make informed decisions about your training program, allowing you to progress safely and effectively toward your fitness goals.

Balancing Core Work with Other Fitness Activities

While core training is essential for developing a strong and functional midsection, it's important to balance your core work with other fitness activities to ensure a well-rounded approach to fitness. Here's how to strike the right balance:

- **Incorporate Strength Training**: In addition to core-specific exercises, incorporate full-body strength training into your routine to build overall strength and muscle mass. Compound exercises such as squats, deadlifts, rows, and presses engage multiple muscle groups simultaneously, including the core, and help improve functional strength and stability.

- **Include Cardiovascular Exercise**: Cardiovascular exercise is essential for heart health, calorie burn, and overall fitness. Incorporate activities such as running, cycling, swimming, or HIIT workouts into your routine to improve cardiovascular endurance and support fat loss.

- **Prioritize Flexibility and Mobility**: Flexibility and mobility are often overlooked aspects of fitness but are crucial for injury prevention and overall well-being. Incorporate flexibility exercises such as yoga, Pilates, or stretching into your routine to improve flexibility, mobility, and joint health.

- **Listen to Your Body**: As always, listen to your body and adjust your training program accordingly. If you're feeling fatigued or overworked, scale back the intensity or volume of your workouts, or take an extra rest day. Prioritize recovery and give your body the time it needs to rest and repair.

By incorporating a variety of activities into your fitness routine, you'll ensure a well-rounded approach to fitness that supports overall health, strength, and function. Remember to listen to your body, prioritize recovery, and strike the right balance between core work and other fitness activities to achieve your fitness goals safely and effectively.

avoiding common mistakes in core training requires a combination of awareness, mindfulness, and balance. By avoiding overtraining and injury, listening to your body's signals, and balancing core work with other fitness activities, you'll set yourself up for success in your fitness journey. Remember to progress gradually, prioritize recovery, and listen to what your body is telling you to achieve your core strength and fitness goals safely and effectively.

STAYING MOTIVATED

Maintaining motivation is often the key factor that determines whether you succeed in your fitness journey or fall short of your goals. In this chapter, we'll explore strategies for staying motivated, including overcoming procrastination and excuses, finding your source of inspiration, and celebrating small victories and progress along the way.

Overcoming Procrastination and Excuses

Procrastination and excuses are two of the most common barriers that can derail your fitness goals. Whether it's putting off a workout until tomorrow or finding reasons why you can't stick to your nutrition plan, overcoming these obstacles is essential for staying on track and making progress. Here's how to overcome procrastination and excuses:

- **Identify Your Triggers**: Take some time to reflect on what triggers your procrastination and excuses. Are there specific tasks or situations that make you more likely to procrastinate? Are there recurring excuses that you find yourself making to justify skipping workouts or indulging in unhealthy foods? By identifying your triggers, you can develop strategies to address them more effectively.

- **Set Clear Goals**: Having clear, specific goals can help keep you motivated and focused on your fitness journey. Break down your larger goals into smaller, more manageable tasks, and set deadlines for achieving them. This can help prevent overwhelm and make it easier to stay motivated and on track.

- **Create a Routine**: Establishing a consistent routine can help minimize the opportunity for procrastination and excuses. Schedule your workouts and meal prep sessions at the same time each day or week, and stick to your plan as much as possible. Over time, your routine will become a habit, making it easier to stay motivated and avoid procrastination.

- **Hold Yourself Accountable**: Find ways to hold yourself accountable for your actions and progress. This could involve tracking your workouts and nutrition in a journal or app, sharing your goals with a friend or family member for support, or joining a fitness community or group to stay motivated and accountable.

- **Practice Self-Compassion**: It's important to remember that everyone struggles with procrastination and excuses from time to time, and that's okay. Instead of beating yourself up when you slip up, practice self-compassion and focus on moving forward. Learn from your mistakes, make adjustments as needed, and keep pushing towards your goals.

By identifying your triggers, setting clear goals, establishing a routine, holding yourself accountable, and practicing self-compassion, you can overcome procrastination and excuses and stay motivated on your fitness journey.

Finding Your Source of Inspiration

Finding your source of inspiration can help fuel your motivation and keep you committed to your fitness goals, even when the going gets tough. Whether it's a role model, a personal goal, or a deeper purpose, having something to inspire you can make all the difference in staying motivated. Here's how to find your source of inspiration:

- **Identify Your Why**: Take some time to reflect on why you want to improve your health and fitness. What are your underlying reasons and motivations? Is it to feel more confident in your body, improve your overall health, or set a positive example for your loved ones? Understanding your why can help fuel your motivation and keep you focused on your goals.

- **Find Role Models**: Look for people who inspire you and embody the qualities or achievements you aspire to. Whether it's a fitness influencer, a professional athlete, or a friend or family member who has achieved their fitness goals, surrounding yourself with positive role models can help keep you motivated and inspired on your own journey.

- **Visualize Success**: Take some time each day to visualize yourself achieving your fitness goals. Imagine how you'll look, feel, and move when you've reached your desired level of health and fitness. Visualizing success can help reinforce your motivation and keep you focused on your goals, even when faced with challenges or setbacks.

- **Set Meaningful Goals**: Set goals that are personally meaningful and aligned with your values and priorities. Instead of focusing solely on aesthetics or external validation, consider setting goals that reflect your desire for health, vitality, and overall well-being. This can help ensure that your motivation remains intrinsic and enduring, rather than fleeting and superficial.

- **Seek Inspiration Everywhere**: Inspiration can be found in the most unexpected places. Stay open to new experiences, perspectives, and opportunities for growth, and seek inspiration in the world around you. Whether it's a beautiful sunrise, a powerful quote, or a meaningful conversation with a friend, finding inspiration in everyday moments can help keep your motivation alive and well.

By identifying your why, finding role models, visualizing success, setting meaningful goals, and seeking inspiration everywhere, you can find your source of inspiration and fuel your motivation to achieve your fitness goals.

Celebrating Small Victories and Progress

Celebrating small victories and progress along the way is essential for maintaining motivation and momentum on your fitness journey. While it's natural to focus on the end goal, taking the time to acknowledge and celebrate your achievements along the way can help keep you motivated and inspired. Here's how to celebrate small victories and progress:

- **Acknowledge Your Achievements**: Take a moment to acknowledge and celebrate your achievements, no matter how small they may seem. Whether it's completing a challenging workout, making healthier food choices, or sticking to your plan despite obstacles or setbacks, every step forward is worth celebrating.

- **Keep a Progress Journal**: Keep a journal or log of your progress, including achievements, milestones, and moments of growth. This can help you track your progress over time and provide a visual reminder of how far you've come. Reviewing your progress journal regularly can help boost your confidence and motivation, especially during times of doubt or frustration.

- **Reward Yourself**: Treat yourself to a reward or indulgence as a way of celebrating your achievements. Whether it's a massage, a new workout outfit, or a special meal, choose rewards that are meaningful and aligned with your goals. This can help reinforce positive behaviors and provide added motivation to continue making progress.

- **Share Your Successes**: Don't be afraid to share your successes with others and celebrate your achievements together. Whether it's sharing a post on social media, telling a friend or family member, or joining a fitness community or group, sharing your successes can help amplify your sense of accomplishment and inspire others along the way.

- **Reflect on Your Growth**: Take some time to reflect on how far you've come and the progress you've made on your fitness journey. Recognize the obstacles you've overcome, the lessons you've learned, and the strength and resilience you've developed along the way. Reflecting on your growth can help cultivate a sense of gratitude and appreciation for your journey and fuel your motivation to keep moving forward.

By acknowledging your achievements, keeping a progress journal, rewarding yourself, sharing your successes, and reflecting on your growth, you can celebrate small victories and progress along the way and stay motivated on your fitness journey.

staying motivated on your fitness journey requires a combination of awareness, inspiration, and celebration. By overcoming procrastination and excuses, finding your source of inspiration, and celebrating small victories and progress along the way, you can stay motivated and committed to achieving your health and fitness goals. Remember to stay focused on your why, surround yourself with positive influences, and celebrate every step forward, no matter how small. With determination, perseverance, and a positive mindset, you can stay motivated and achieve your fitness goals.

FAQS AND TROUBLESHOOTING

In this chapter, we'll address common questions and concerns related to core exercise, troubleshoot common issues that may arise during your training, and discuss when it may be necessary to seek professional guidance. Whether you're a beginner or experienced exerciser, understanding these FAQs and troubleshooting tips can help you navigate your core training journey more effectively.

Addressing Common Questions and Concerns

- **Do I Need Equipment to Train My Core?** While equipment such as stability balls, resistance bands, and weights can add variety and intensity to your core workouts, they're not strictly necessary. Many effective core exercises can be done using only your body weight, such as planks, crunches, and leg raises. However, incorporating equipment can help challenge your muscles in new ways and add variety to your routine.

- **How Often Should I Train My Core?** The frequency of your core training will depend on your goals, fitness level, and overall workout routine. For most people, training the core 2-3 times per week is sufficient to see results. However, it's essential to listen to your body and allow for adequate rest and recovery between sessions.

- **Can I Train My Core Every Day?** While it's tempting to train your core every day in hopes of faster results, overtraining can lead to burnout, fatigue, and increased risk of injury. It's essential to give your core muscles time to rest and recover between workouts to allow for proper repair and growth. Aim to include at least one or two rest days per week to prevent overtraining.

- **How Long Does It Take to See Results?** The time it takes to see results from core training will vary depending on factors such as your starting fitness level, consistency, and adherence to proper form and technique. With consistent effort and dedication, you can expect to see improvements in core strength, stability, and appearance within a few weeks to a few months.

- **What Are the Best Core Exercises for Beginners?** For beginners, it's best to start with simple, foundational exercises that target the major muscle groups of the core. Examples include planks, crunches, bicycle crunches, and leg raises. These exercises are relatively easy to perform and can help build a strong foundation of core strength and stability.

- **How Can I Prevent Neck or Back Pain During Core Exercises?** Neck or back pain during core exercises is often a sign of poor form or technique. To prevent pain and injury, focus on maintaining a neutral spine position throughout the exercise, engage your core muscles to support your back, and avoid straining your neck by keeping your gaze forward or slightly upward.

- **Should I Include Cardiovascular Exercise in My Core Training Routine?** While core exercises primarily target the muscles of the midsection, cardiovascular exercise is essential for overall health and fitness. Including cardio workouts such as running, cycling, swimming, or HIIT can help improve cardiovascular endurance, burn calories, and support fat loss, which can enhance the visibility of your core muscles.

Troubleshooting Common Core Exercise Issues

- **Feeling Neck or Back Strain**: If you're experiencing neck or back strain during core exercises, it's essential to check your form and technique. Focus on maintaining a neutral spine position, engage your core muscles to support your back, and avoid straining your neck by keeping your gaze forward or slightly upward. If pain persists, consider modifying the exercise or seeking guidance from a fitness professional.

- **Difficulty Maintaining Balance**: Balance can be a common issue during core exercises, especially for beginners. To improve balance, focus on engaging your core muscles to stabilize your body, start with simpler exercises and progress gradually to more challenging variations, and practice mindfulness and focus during your workouts. Additionally, incorporating balance training exercises such as single-leg stands or stability ball exercises can help improve balance and stability over time.

- **Lack of Progress or Plateau**: If you've hit a plateau or are struggling to see progress in your core training, it may be time to shake up your routine. Try incorporating new exercises, increasing the intensity or volume of your workouts, or varying the tempo or duration of your exercises. Additionally, focusing on proper form and technique, ensuring adequate rest and recovery, and addressing any nutritional or lifestyle factors that may be impacting your progress can help break through plateaus and see continued improvements.

- **Feeling Disengaged or Bored**: If you're feeling disengaged or bored with your core training routine, it's essential to keep things fresh and exciting. Try incorporating new exercises, challenging yourself with different variations or equipment, or mixing up the order or timing of your workouts. Additionally, setting new goals, tracking your progress, and celebrating small victories along the way can help keep you motivated and engaged in your training.

- **Experiencing Muscle Imbalances**: Muscle imbalances can occur when certain muscles become stronger or tighter than others, leading to poor posture, movement dysfunction, and increased risk of injury. To address muscle imbalances, focus on incorporating exercises that target both the front and back of the core, as well as the sides, to ensure balanced development. Additionally, incorporating unilateral exercises (those that work one side of the body at a time) and stretching tight muscles can help restore balance and symmetry to your core muscles.

Seeking Professional Guidance When Necessary

While many common core exercise issues can be addressed through self-awareness, proper technique, and troubleshooting, there may be times when it's necessary to seek professional guidance. Here are some situations where seeking guidance from a fitness professional or healthcare provider may be beneficial:

- **Persistent Pain or Discomfort**: If you're experiencing persistent pain or discomfort during core exercises, it's essential to listen to your body and seek guidance from a qualified fitness professional or healthcare provider. They can assess your form and technique, identify any underlying issues or imbalances, and provide personalized recommendations for modifying your workouts to prevent further injury.

- **Difficulty Progressing or Seeing Results**: If you're struggling to progress in your core training or are not seeing the results you desire; it may be helpful to consult with a fitness professional or personal trainer. They can assess your current fitness level, evaluate your training program, and provide expert guidance on how to modify your workouts, set realistic goals, and achieve optimal results.

- **Concerns About Form or Technique**: If you're unsure whether you're performing core exercises correctly or have concerns about your form or technique, seeking guidance from a qualified fitness professional or personal trainer can provide valuable feedback and support. They can assess your form, offer corrections and modifications as needed, and ensure that you're performing exercises safely and effectively to minimize the risk of injury.

- **Nutritional or Lifestyle Concerns**: If you have questions or concerns about nutrition, hydration, sleep, or other lifestyle factors that may be impacting your core training, consulting with a registered dietitian, nutritionist, or healthcare provider can provide valuable insight and guidance. They can assess your current habits, offer personalized recommendations for improving your nutrition and lifestyle, and help you create a plan that supports your fitness goals and overall well-being.

addressing common questions and concerns, troubleshooting common core exercise issues, and seeking professional guidance when necessary are essential components of a successful core training program. By understanding how to overcome common challenges, adjust your approach as needed, and seek support when necessary, you can navigate your core training journey more effectively and achieve your health and fitness goals safely and efficiently. Remember to listen to your body, prioritize proper form and technique, and be proactive in seeking guidance and support when needed to ensure a positive and rewarding fitness experience.

BEYOND 5 MINUTES: ADVANCED CORE CHALLENGES

In this chapter, we'll delve into advanced strategies for taking your core training to the next level. We'll explore longer core workouts, integrating core exercises into full-body workouts, and setting new goals and challenges to keep your progress moving forward.

When you're ready to push past the limitations of a 5-minute routine and challenge your core muscles in new ways, these advanced techniques will help you maximize your strength, stability, and overall fitness.

Exploring Longer Core Workouts

While 5-minute core workouts are a great way to build consistency and establish a foundation of strength, advancing beyond this timeframe can provide additional benefits and challenges for your core muscles.

When exploring longer core workouts, it's important to focus on quality over quantity. Instead of simply extending the duration of your exercises, aim to incorporate a variety of movements and techniques that target different areas of your core and challenge your muscles in new ways. Consider incorporating exercises such as:

- Plank variations (side planks, plank with leg lifts, plank with shoulder taps)
- Dynamic movements (mountain climbers, Russian twists, bicycle crunches)
- Isometric holds (boat pose, hollow hold, dead bug)

By mixing and matching these exercises and adjusting the duration and intensity to suit your fitness level, you can create a longer core workout that provides a comprehensive challenge for your core muscles while also promoting endurance, stability, and functional strength.

When designing longer core workouts, be sure to include proper warm-up and cool-down periods to prepare your body for exercise and promote recovery afterward. Incorporating dynamic stretches, mobility exercises, and foam rolling can help improve circulation, reduce muscle tension, and enhance overall performance and recovery.

Integrating Core Exercises into Full-Body Workouts

In addition to standalone core workouts, integrating core exercises into full-body workouts can help maximize your training efficiency and effectiveness while also promoting balanced muscle development and functional movement patterns.

When incorporating core exercises into full-body workouts, consider the following tips:

1. **Compound Movements**: Choose compound exercises that engage multiple muscle groups simultaneously, such as squats, deadlifts, lunges, and overhead presses. These exercises require core stability and strength to maintain proper form and alignment, making them excellent choices for integrating core work into your routine.

2. **Circuit Training**: Structure your workouts as circuits, alternating between strength exercises for different muscle groups and core exercises to keep your heart rate elevated and maximize calorie burn. Aim to include a mix of upper body, lower body, and core exercises in each circuit to provide a comprehensive full-body workout.

3. **Functional Movement Patterns**: Select core exercises that mimic real-life movements and activities to improve functional strength and mobility. Exercises such as farmer's carries, bear crawls, and kettlebell swings challenge your core muscles in dynamic, multi-directional ways, helping improve stability, coordination, and athletic performance.

4. **Balance and Stability Training**: Incorporate balance and stability exercises into your workouts to challenge your core muscles in new ways and improve proprioception and body awareness. Exercises such as single-leg deadlifts, stability ball rollouts, and plank variations on unstable surfaces require core engagement to maintain balance and stability, making them effective additions to full-body workouts.

By integrating core exercises into full-body workouts, you can maximize your training efficiency and effectiveness while also promoting balanced muscle development, functional movement patterns, and overall fitness.

Setting New Goals and Challenges

As you progress in your core training journey, it's essential to continually set new goals and challenges to keep your workouts fresh, exciting, and effective. Whether you've mastered the basics or are ready to take your core strength to the next level, setting new goals can help keep you motivated and engaged in your training.

When setting new goals and challenges for your core training, consider the following tips:

1. **Progressive Overload**: Gradually increase the intensity, volume, or complexity of your core exercises to continually challenge

your muscles and promote growth and adaptation. This could involve increasing the weight, reps, or duration of your exercises, or incorporating advanced variations and techniques to keep your workouts challenging and effective.

2. **Specificity**: Set specific, measurable, and achievable goals that are tailored to your individual needs and priorities. Whether your goal is to improve core strength, stability, endurance, or aesthetics, having a clear objective will help guide your training and keep you focused on making progress.

3. **Variety and Diversity**: Incorporate a variety of exercises, techniques, and training modalities into your core workouts to keep your muscles guessing and prevent stagnation. Experiment with different exercises, equipment, and training methods to challenge your core muscles in new ways and keep your workouts interesting and effective.

4. **Long-Term Vision**: Keep the big picture in mind and focus on long-term progress and growth rather than short-term results. Set realistic expectations for yourself and understand that achieving significant improvements in core strength and aesthetics takes time, consistency, and dedication. Celebrate small victories along the way and trust in the process of continuous improvement.

By setting new goals and challenges, you can keep your core training journey exciting, motivating, and rewarding, while also ensuring that you continue to make progress and achieve your fitness goals.

In conclusion, advancing beyond 5-minute core workouts requires a strategic approach that includes exploring longer core workouts, integrating core exercises into full-body workouts, and setting new goals and challenges to keep your progress moving forward. By incorporating these advanced techniques into your training regimen, you can maximize your core strength, stability, and overall fitness, while also enjoying the benefits of a strong and functional midsection. Remember to listen to your body, progress gradually, and stay committed to your goals, and you'll be well on your way to achieving the strong, healthy core you desire.

CONCLUSION

In conclusion, the journey through core exercise has been a comprehensive exploration of not just physical fitness, but also holistic well-being. From the basics of getting started and understanding core anatomy to advancing into more challenging workouts and addressing common pitfalls, we've traversed the landscape of core strength and stability with diligence and purpose.

Throughout this journey, we've uncovered the multitude of benefits that core exercise offers. Beyond the aesthetic appeal of sculpted abs, core training improves posture, enhances balance, boosts athletic performance, reduces the risk of injury, and promotes functional fitness in everyday life. Whether you're a seasoned athlete striving for peak performance or an individual seeking to lead a healthier, more active lifestyle, core exercise is an essential component of any well-rounded fitness regimen.

But beyond the physical benefits lies a deeper truth: the journey to a strong and resilient core is a reflection of the journey to overall health and vitality. It requires commitment, perseverance, and a willingness to push past comfort zones and embrace challenges. It's about cultivating not just physical strength, but also mental fortitude, emotional resilience, and spiritual well-being.

As you continue on your journey of self-improvement and personal growth, remember that health is not just the absence of illness, but the presence of vitality and vigor in every aspect of your life. It's about nourishing your body, mind, and soul with wholesome foods, positive thoughts, and meaningful connections. It's about embracing movement as a celebration of what your body can do, rather than a punishment for what it's not.

In the words of the renowned naturalist and essayist John Muir, "The clearest way into the Universe is through a forest wilderness." Just as exploring the depths of nature opens our eyes to the wonders of the universe, so too does embarking on the journey of health and fitness open our hearts to the infinite possibilities of our own potential.

So, dear reader, I encourage you to embrace the journey with open arms and a steadfast resolve. Embrace the challenges, celebrate the victories, and never lose sight of the incredible resilience and strength that lies within you. For in the pursuit of health and vitality, the greatest rewards are not found at the destination, but in the journey itself.